MW01074665

Published in the UK by Bruckshaw Media
Cover design by Mohamed Mustapha and Pete Bruckshaw
Layout design by Pete Bruckshaw

Edition One

**Looking Amazing And Feeling Great
Has Never Been Easier...**

**"Free Rapid Fat-Loss Cheatsheet
Reveals The Simple 7-Step System
That Fast Tracks You To Your Ideal
Weight — And Keeps You There!"**

Visit This Link For Your Free Gift:

http://bruckshawdiet.com/gift

Thank You...

To all my family for their invaluable support over the years.

Thanks also to Christopher John Payne. Chris was there all the way for me with invaluable advice on the content and presentation of this book. Chris's website is www.christopherjohnpayne.com

And most importantly, this book is dedicated to the memory of my parents, who both passed away recently; to my Mum for her encouragement and to my Dad for his inspiration.

Contents

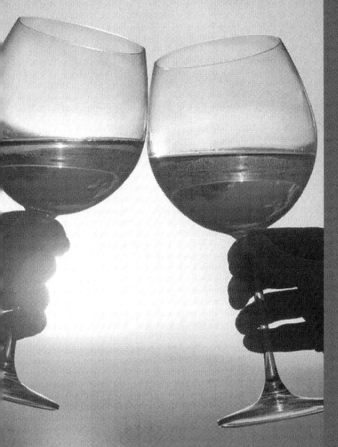

chapter **1**

24 Hours To Success

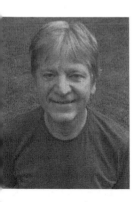

Pete Bruckshaw here with a headstart for you on The Wine Drinker's Diet. It's time for 24 Hours To Success.

In the words of Benjamin Franklin...

"Those that fail to plan, plan to fail."

That's why I'm going to give you a unique system that will get you off to the best possible start. I'll guide you smoothly through the first twenty-four crucial hours of your diet.

These step-by-step instructions are unlike anything you've ever read in a diet book before.

I'll urge you on as you head towards your weight loss goals. Once you've successfully finished your first twenty-four hours of the Wine Drinker's Diet, you'll know that you *can* do this!

In 24 Hours To Success I don't just tell you *what* to do. I show you *how* to do it!

If you're like me you've read more than your share of diet books. But if they worked you wouldn't be reading this now.

I love my food — and drink. I'm not loaded with will power. Despite that **I lost weight and kept it off.**

But really, that's just me.

And whilst I've spent most of my life overweight, I've never been obese. If that's you, you'll have to work longer and harder to reach your ideal weight.

So can I guarantee your success?

The short answer is... NO.

Because there isn't a magic diet pill. Or a quick fix solution. And I don't know you or what you're capable of.

But I know this much: With The 24 Hour Success System your chances of winning with The Wine Drinker's Diet will increase *dramatically*.

For years I dreamt of meeting my weight loss goals. But it just became more of a struggle. The more frustrated I got, the more I ate.

But I read up. Talked to the right people. And I wised up.

My knowledge and experience enabled me to develop The Wine Drinker's Diet.

Are your ready to live longer? Are you ready to look and feel better than you have done in years?

Then let's get started with 24 Hours To Success.

First of all, it's vital to choose the right time to begin. Start at 7 pm. Make sure you're away from work for the following day. For most working people this is best begun on a Friday night.

1. Share The Wine Drinkers Diet

The first rule of the 24 Hour Success System is this:

Make Yourself Accountable.

The most important people to tell are those that you share your daily living space with. So whether that's your girlfriend, boyfriend, spouse, family, friends... you *need* to talk to them about The Wine Drinker's Diet. I hope that they will actively encourage you in your weight loss goals.

Unfortunately those closest to us can sometimes be less supportive than we want them to be.

But don't let them discourage you this time! Determine that you'll show them how you're going to make The Wine Drinker's Diet work for you.

Keep reading to find out why living on your own makes this system much easier for you to succeed with.

Regardless of whether you have support for your diet goals or not, you're still accountable to the people you confide in.

This is how to do it:

Show your loved ones your copy of The Wine Drinker's Diet. Explain that you are going to eat well but wisely. Invite them to join you in clearing the cupboards of stodgy sugar and fat laden food. Offer to cook everyone the same food that you're planning to eat.

Finding a diet buddy is another way to increase your chances of success with The Wine Drinker's Diet.

If you know someone who can stand to lose a pound or two, they may want to join you to meet their own diet goals. Guide them through the highlights of the book, be your usual tactful self, and explain how it will be easier for both of you if you do this together.

Conversely, some of your loved ones may have no intention of joining you on your journey. Find their favourite foods in The Wine Drinker's Diet and explain that you will be including them in your meals. And if they want larger portions than you'll be eating, why complain?

Remember that this is all good healthy nutritious food. It's the kind that you can comfortably feed your family with.

If you do live on your own, you can still tell your loved ones about the diet you're starting. Tell them that you're making yourself accountable to them. Next time you talk to them, tell them exactly how you're doing with The Wine Drinker's Diet.

If you take meals or snacks with your co-workers, they need to be told about The Wine Drinker's Diet too. But you can do that later. For now we'll concentrate on getting you successfully through the first 24 hours of The Wine Drinker's Diet.

2. Blitz Your Kitchen Cupboards

You need to clean your kitchen out of any forbidden food that will tempt you to break your diet.

If you have the strength to take or leave fatty or sugar laden food, that's fine.

But the rest of us need to avoid the temptation that well-stocked food cupboards can bring.

Instant food that requires no preparation is best avoided. Crisps, cereal, biscuits and cake are the worst offenders.

The best option is to throw out any food that will tempt you. If you're on your own it's easiest of all. Keeping your shelves stocked with food that's part of this diet is the ideal you should aim for.

But if you live with anyone who will crucify you if you throw away the biscuits and crisps, try to reach a compromise. Find a place for them to store their food that won't tempt you constantly. Then you'll both be happy with the arrangement.

Identify flashpoints when your will is at its weakest. Then you can deal with them before they happen.

For instance I can easily avoid attacking the cupboards if I follow The Wine Drinker's Diet during the daytime. But during the evenings I have to be careful.

For these times keep some snacks close at hand. Carrots cut into batons work well for me.

And if you need a protein top up between meals an extra boiled egg won't hurt either.

So what are you going to replace all that empty cupboard and fridge space with? Keep reading...

3. Enjoy Your Meals

Go to Chapter Seven in this book. Now choose what you want to eat for the first day of your diet. Buy the food in if you haven't done already. If you need to, remember to get extra so that you can cook some for your loved ones too.

And don't forget your drink either. Get your day's allowance ready beforehand. If you'll be tempted to drink more, make sure that you only have your daily allowance on hand.

Now have a good night's sleep and get ready to begin your diet tomorrow.

Start the day early with the recommended exercises from The Wine Drinker's Diet in Chapter Five. If you're able to, the best time to exercise is before anyone else gets up, first thing in the morning.

For breakfast and lunch, follow your meal instructions again in Chapter Seven.

For your main meal don't forget to include a glass or two of wine (you probably don't need to be reminded!).

4. Drink To Your Success!

And after the meal why not take a brandy to round it off? Or perhaps another glass of wine?

Cheers!

You've made it through the first day of The Wine Drinker's Diet.

You've bought this book. You're reading this chapter. And you know that if you really apply what I show you, you'll achieve incredible results.

If you've found this chapter helpful I recommend my Slim For Life programme.

To find out more visit the link below.

http://bruckshawdiet.com/sfl.html

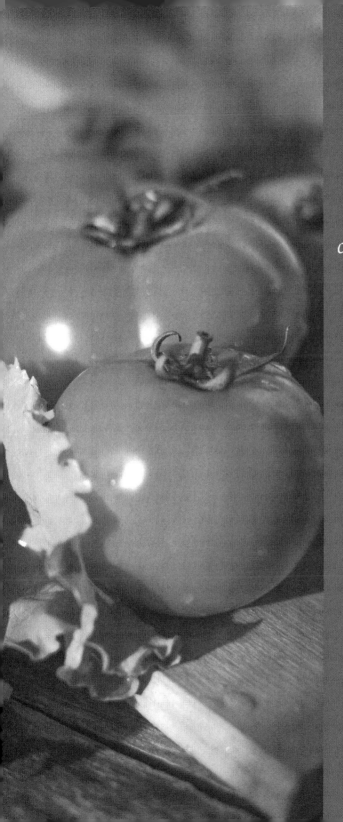

chapter **2**

Why I Created The Wine Drinker's Diet

Most of my life I've been overweight. Sometimes a little. Sometimes a lot more. But I never dealt with the problem. And it got worse.

I'm Pete Bruckshaw. I've spent most of my adult life either putting weight on or trying to lose it. Is wanting to be slim a vanity thing?

Maybe.

But as I've become older I've seen friends and family putting weight on and suffering because of it. Some have gone before their time — directly as a result of their weight problems.

Losing weight isn't just about looking good. For many of us it becomes a matter of life and death.

For me it's something I desperately needed to deal with. And the problem was there every time a looked in the mirror.

This is my story...

My wife is a civil servant, and her job has meant that we've done our fair share of travelling outside the UK.

When I was in my 40s I lived with my wife and daughter in Belgium.

I've always associated countries with the food and drink indigenous to them.

So Belgium means plenty of rich chocolates, crispy fries smeared with mayonnaise...

And beer. Belgian beer is some of the best in the world. It's powerful at up to 12% strength. But traditional Belgian beer is 100% naturally brewed. A taste sensation with a kick to match. Unlike the chemical cosh you'd expect from a similarly strong British lager.

I felt obliged — no, duty bound — to make a large dent in the three hundred plus different Belgian beers while I was there.

Needless to say the chocolate, fries and beer diet didn't do much for my waistline.

At 16 stone (224 lbs) I was grossly overweight. And worse still, I had accepted it. When I looked around I took cold comfort from the obese regulars at the local fast food joints (to which my visits were frequent); compared to them I didn't seem so fat. But I *knew* I needed to sort myself out. Finally I had to lose weight.

I tried a low fat diet. That meant constant calorie counting and eating and drinking less of everything I liked. It was tough. But I kept at it. A month later I was four pounds down.

The problem was that I resented the borderline starvation I was putting myself through. I started treating myself to the occasional burger at McDonalds. Those were the days of Supersize meals. Why not go large? I'd deal with the guilt later.

And one or two of those beers wouldn't hurt, would they? And maybe a couple more for luck... Just as quickly the pounds piled back on.

I was back where I started. Again.

Could more exercise be the answer?

I joined my local gym. A trainer showed me the exercises I needed to do to lose weight and get in shape. I worked out three times a week.

My muscle tone and fitness level definitely improved. But there was a catch.

After each workout I craved food. I *deserved* food after all that exercise! I ended up putting that lost weight right back on again.

What I really wanted was a diet for life. A diet with food that I enjoyed and treats in moderation. I wanted to keep fit too. And wanted a few drinks when I felt like it. All without going overboard and sabotaging my diet goals.

The harder I tried the more difficult losing weight seemed to be. At the point when I was resigning myself to being fat forever, I discovered a diet system that worked for me.

On a visit back to the UK, I went to my doctor to see what he would recommend. There are plenty of doctors who would have told me to take up the kind of low fat diet that had already failed for me.

Fortunately I was in luck. My doctor drew up a low carbohydrate diet plan. This was a whole new way of dieting for me.

The diet was straightforward enough.

Plenty of protein: lots of meals based on meat, fish and eggs. No processed carbs. I binned the cereals, white bread and biscuits.

I began exercising 10 minutes a day. Nothing too strenuous. Just sit ups, press ups and stomach crunches. Now I wasn't working up a sweat and getting hungry. Instead my fitness and well being improved. My posture was better. Everything fitted in perfectly with my weight loss plan.

The weight fell off me over the next three months. I went from 16 stone (224 lbs) to 13 stone 10 lbs (192 lbs). I became a dieting obsessive. I kept on studying for more information.

My target weight was 12 stone 12 lbs (181 lbs).

And here I discovered a flaw with the low carb diet. Despite maintaining the same regime, my weight had plateaud. There was no shifting those extra pounds. I lost confidence in myself and the diet. I still practiced it – just about — but I put on a few lbs, hit 14 stone (196 lbs) and pretty much stayed there for the following year.

Decision time. I didn't want to stay overweight forever. It was time to take matters into my own hands. I wanted to create a diet that worked long term for me and other people too.

One of the things I enjoyed was a morning fry up: bacon, sausages and black pudding. This is a staple of low carb diets. Only thing is I didn't actually *need* that food. Like most westerners I live a fairly sedentary lifestyle. So I ditched the big breakfast.

Providing I kept the cupboard and fridge shelves reasonably clear, I was surprised to find that I could survive and thrive on just a boiled egg for breakfast and one for lunch. After a couple of years of daily fry ups I thought I would be starving. But because eggs are filling as well as nutrition-packed that was not the case.

A couple of snacks, say carrots or yoghurt, would keep me going too. My hunger pangs would only really strike in the evening.

And this is when I ate a generous meal of fish or lean meat and vegetables. Always grilled or steamed. Never fried.

I started to vary my protein intake during the day. And the weight was starting to come off.

Gaining in confidence, I decided to work in a few more things that the doctor *didn't* order. Would it be possible to re-introduce alcoholic drinks and still keep the weight off?

It would.

Cautiously at first I added food and drink that I'd previously enjoyed. I followed simple guidelines. For the most part I avoided sugar and processed carbohydrates (give or take the occasional treat). I rarely drank beer because of the high sugar and carbohydrate content.

Saving the big meal for the evening had another significant effect too. I found that I could enjoy wine before, during and after my meal and still lose weight!

To combat the munchies that often strike when you enjoy a tipple or two I would sometimes keep a little of my meal back for supper.

I reached my ideal 12 stone 12 lbs weight (180 lbs) — and the pounds stayed off.

I created a varied and achievable diet for life. A diet that lets you enjoy the good things in life while you lose weight and get healthy: The Wine Drinker's Diet.

This diet is designed for just about everybody. You don't need to drink to do it! Of course if you're teetotal you'll lose weight on this diet even faster.

Most of the high protein in this diet is from meat, fish and eggs. But vegetarians can still lose weight on The Wine Drinker's Diet. I include meat-free recipes throughout the book.

So who is The Wine Drinker's Diet NOT for?

If you're under 18 or are a pregnant or lactating woman you shouldn't be on The Wine Drinker's Diet.

Before starting this diet you should consult your GP. If your physical health is below par The Wine Drinker's Diet may not be suitable for you.

If you think you may have an alcohol problem The Wine Drinker's Diet is not for you either. You need a doctor, not a diet and I recommend you seek advice at the earliest possible opportunity.

But if that's not you, no worries. You're about to be introduced to the only diet you'll ever need.

Are you ready to get slim and STAY slim?

Then join me now on the diet that will change your life forever — The Wine Drinker's Diet.

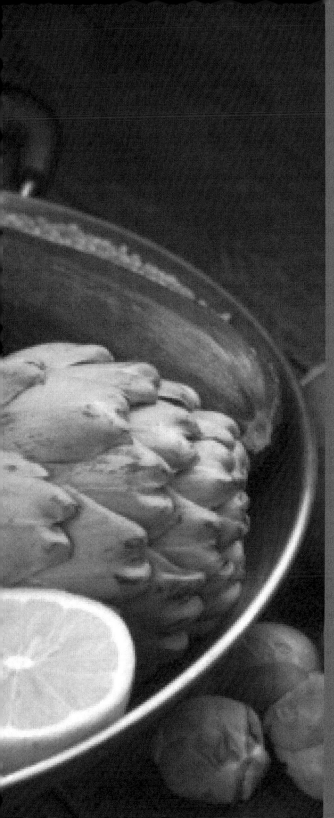

chapter **3**

Wine Is Wonderful

Numerous studies bear out what you probably knew already: a tincture or two does you the power of good. Here's the latest news...

Wine And Weight Loss: A Great Combination

Wine is a good option for dieters because it has far less carbohydrates than beer. It's also low in sugar providing you avoid sweet white wines.

Why Wine Might Have The Edge On Exercise

A survey conducted by the University of Alberta in Canada found that the resveratrol found in wine improves physical and mental functions in a similar way to a workout at the gym.

Whilst resveratrol is present in all wine, it's most concentrated in red wine.

Live Longer With Wine

A Harvard Medical School study reports that the combination of resveratrol and the SIRT1 gene (which also occurs in red wine) is linked to longer life and better health.

Drink To A Healthy Heart

A study for the European IMMIDIET project concluded that wine is the best drink for improving your omega-3 levels. Increasing these fatty acids means more protection for you against coronary heart disease.

Wine Can Reduce Liver Disease

An excess of any alcohol can cause alcoholic fatty liver disease. But a study by the UC San Diego School of Medicine reports that wine taken regularly in moderation is the only drink that can reduce the risk of non-alcoholic fatty liver disease by up to 50%. In contrast beer and spirit drinkers have over four times the risk of non-alcoholic fatty liver disease than wine drinkers.

Chase Your Blues Away

Research from Spain for the BMC Medicine journal reports that two to seven glasses of red wine a week can decrease depression. Even when lifestyle factors are taken into account the results are the same.

So let's drink to a healthier lifestyle! But before you get started on this life changing diet I'll deal with some frequently asked questions.

chapter **4**

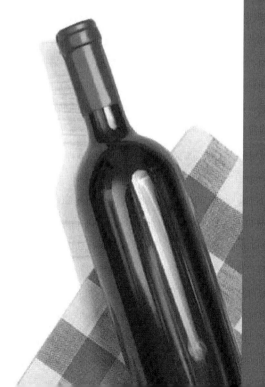

Questions
And Answers

I'm sure you're keen to get started with this fast weight loss system. But maybe you want to know more first. Here I'll answer the questions that I'm often asked about The Wine Drinker's Diet.

How does The Wine Drinker's Diet work?

The induction phase is Level One of The Wine Drinker's Diet. It lasts just one week.

During the first week, you'll detox your body. You won't be starving yourself; you'll never go hungry on this diet.

Instead you'll cut out processed foods and sugar. You'll learn a new way of eating.

Most westerners lead sedentary lives. There's no need to bulk up on a big cooked meal to start the day. Instead you'll take a light breakfast and lunch.

For years I've started the day with a full cooked fried breakfast. I was surprised how easy it was for me to eat far less and still not be hungry during the daytime.

The Wine Drinker's Diet is ideal if you like a drink or two during the evening. Feel free to enjoy a glass of wine with your main meal at dinner time. You will soak up some of the alcohol with the meal you eat. And you'll avoid the dreaded munchies — the tendency to attack whatever food is available.

Follow my recommendation and keep a little of your meal back for supper. Think ahead, stay in control and you'll have no problem succeeding with The Wine Drinker's Diet.

Cravings for sweet and fatty foods will begin to diminish as a result. And those pounds will start to fall off.

Stay on Level One for as long as you like. But I recommend just a week if it's too intense for you.

You will continue to lose weight on Level Two. But the process will be slower.

On Level Two we'll introduce naturally lower fat cheese into your diet. This is an ideal way to vary your sources of protein and healthy carbs.

Fruit is back on the menu — low sugar varieties only.

Level Three is your diet for life. It's for when you've reached your ideal weight, want to maintain it and still want a treat or two from time to time.

This is at heart a simple and staightforward diet. I'll repeat some of the essential information as we continue so that The Wine Drinker's Diet is all the more easier for you to follow and succeed with.

What drinks apart from wine can I have?

Whilst red, dry white wine and rosé are low in carbohydrates and sugar, beer is high in both.

That's why you should avoid standard beer altogether. However, a couple of bottles of light beer are fine. The rules relax as you progress with The Wine Drinker's Diet.

Spirits are better news, since they contain no carbohydrates. Choose still or fizzy mineral water to dilute spirits rather than mixers. Most mixer drinks contain sugar or sweetener, so you should avoid them.

Can I use sweetener instead of sugar?

Your body has difficulty telling the difference between sugar and sweetener.

Sugar substitutes mimic the effects of sugar so that blood sugar level rises in the same way with sweeteners as it does with sugar.

Studies have also shown that artificial sweeteners may cause brain damage. Some, such as aspartane, may well do more harm than good.

And we want to keep sugar levels down and avoid the highs and lows that come with large amounts of sugar. Excessive amounts of refined carbohydrates create similar spikes and crashes. Putting your body on a rollercoaster ride is not helpful with efficient weight loss.

So my advice is to avoid sweeteners and get used to the natural taste of food and drink.

However if that's too big a step for you, use stevia when you need to which is a natural sweetener.

What about dairy products?

On Level One you can take a small amount of skimmed milk in your hot drinks and with porridge. Plain yoghurt, ideally natural live yoghurt or low fat yoghurt is fine. Other than that dairy products are not allowed. In Levels Two and Three semi-skimmed milk in drinks and with porridge and other dairy based meals and snacks are back on the menu.

What kind of food will I be eating on The Wine Drinker's Diet?

On this diet you'll be sticking to good hearty food like fish, meat and eggs. And there'll be plenty of vegetables; initially lower carb veg like broccoli and carrots.

You need to take your protein from a variety of different sources to stay healthy and slim; that is increasingly a feature of the diet as it progresses.

Later all vegetables are permitted — including high carb potatoes and parsnips too!

You'll be eating real food, that means no processed 'low fat' foods, no ready meals and nothing with any additives. This may seem like a challenge at first, but after a time it's very easy to find natural foods when you're out shopping. They taste a lot better than processed foods too.

I'm a vegetarian? Is this diet for me?

Absolutely! Your progress may be slower because you take in carbs and protein at the same time with a vegetable and pulse based diet. But there's no reason why The Wine Drinker's Diet won't work for you. Each of the three levels includes meals suitable for vegetarians.

Is this a low carb diet or a low fat diet? And are carbs and fat the enemy?

Principally it's low carb. But The Wine Drinker's Diet avoids some of the excesses that you may have found in other low carb diets. Instead it includes some of the principles found on low fat diets too.

You won't be counting calories or carbs. You'll find most of the information you need in the Food And Drink Table at the end of this book. Inevitably the table doesn't include every single food and drink listed.

If what you want to know about isn't there, don't worry. I'll show you a simple internet search method that will get you the information you need in seconds.

I recommend lean white meat such as skinless chicken and pork rather than too much red meat like beef and steak.

Steaming and grilling food is always preferable to frying. It's a cleaner and healthier way to eat.

Low fat diets often include processed carbohydrates, which fill you up in the short term but soon leave you wanting more.

The Wine Drinker's Diet doesn't allow any processed carbs. You'll eat healthy *real* food instead.

The problem with most low carb diets is that when you go slightly overboard with your carb allowance, that's the day ruined.

I'm not discounting carbs or fat. That would lead to an unhealthy diet and illness.

Instead you'll enjoy slow release carbs found in foods like brown rice and oats.

And the natural fat you find in meat can be eaten in moderation on Level Three of The Wine Drinker's Diet.

You'll watch your carb count without being obsessive about it.

You'll eat well without going overboard. Feel free to fill up on protein, ditch the processed carbs, eat less as a result — and lose weight.

The rules are strictest on Level One of The Wine Drinker's Diet.

As this is the fast weight loss stage you want to give yourself as much of an advantage as possible to reach your target weight.

Level One only lasts a week so keep in mind you can look forward to the rules relaxing once you get through the first seven days.

You can still get stuck into sausages, bacon and eggs at the weekend.

And I wouldn't want to live in a world where you can't enjoy a steak with a couple of glasses of wine every now and then. I don't expect you to either!

How much water should I drink?

An ideal amount is about three pints a day. Contrary to some dietary advice you should avoid drinking too much water. It will fill you up but as with everything else water should not be taken to excess. In extreme cases it can cause illness through sodium deficiency.

What about tea and coffee?

Caffeine is a major cause in blood sugar level spikes so I recommend you cut it out completely in Level One.

This can be a shock if you're used to a few hot caffeinated drinks a day. You'll feel tired and listless at first. Remember that this is a sign that your system is becoming cleansed and the diet is working.

These days decaffeinated teas and coffees taste practically the same as drinks with caffeine so you should be able to adjust in that respect.

After Level One, aim to take no more than one caffeinated drink a day.

Having graduated to Level Three I now drink Tetley's English decaffeinated tea most of the time. If I go out somewhere, no sweat, I'll probably end a meal with a caffeinated coffee. A brandy on the side doesn't hurt either!

Doesn't this food involve a lot of preparation?

Not at all. Steaming food is nearly as easy as putting a ready meal in a microwave. And it's a lot healthier too!

How often should I weigh myself?

Twice a week is sufficient. There's no point checking twice a day to see if the pointer on your scales has shifted slightly. Just concentrate on following the diet as much as you can.

And what about the wine?

Treats are in order because the first week is tough. Have one to three glasses of red or dry white wine for five of the seven nights. Or substiture for one to three measures of spirits. See the Food And Drink Table for detailed information.

Of course if you quit drinking, the pounds will fall off all the faster. But you probably didn't buy a book called The Wine Drinker's Diet to be told that!

I assure you that if you follow this diet you can drink and still lose weight. And you'll be fitter and healthier too. How many diets can you say that about?

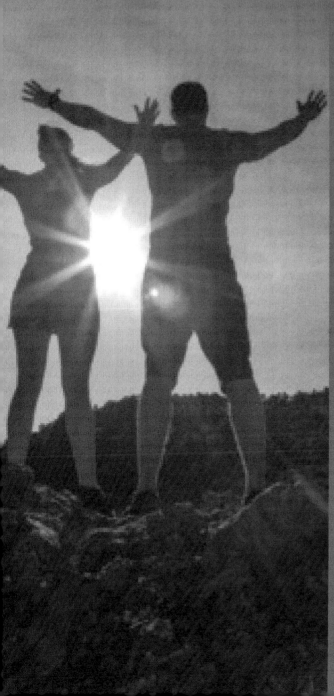

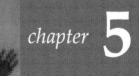

chapter **5**

Exercise

There are some dangerous ideas surrounding modern diets. One is that you don't need to bother exercising on a low carb diet regime. Without exercise on The Wine Drinker's Diet your weight will still decrease fast. But you won't get the same benefits of improved well being, health and physical posture.

I've tried low fat diets that incorporated punishing fitness regimes. I ended up sweating, exhausted — and hungry. As a result I often ended up putting more calories on in food than I lost in exercise.

The Wine Drinker's Diet includes moderate exercise only. Allow yourself a week or so to get in to it. After that time you should be able to stay fit with just twenty minutes a day. Optionally you can double the exercises. But that's not essential. Your main goal is consistency. The minimum you should do these exercises is five days a week. No less.

If it's months or even years since you've exercised then you may need to work up to the exercises more gradually. So start with five of each of the exercises and gradually increase the amount of exercising over the next one - two weeks. Strive for a balance. You should be pushing yourself without getting completely worn out.

The exercises are 25 each of the following:

Star stretches, press ups, alternate leg stretches, stomach crunches, alternate leg raises and cycling.

Star Stretches

These stretches will limber you up before the main exercises. Stretch your arms up in the air above and outwards as far as you can. Put your legs apart and stretch them at the same time. Then relax, stand straight and put your arms by your side.

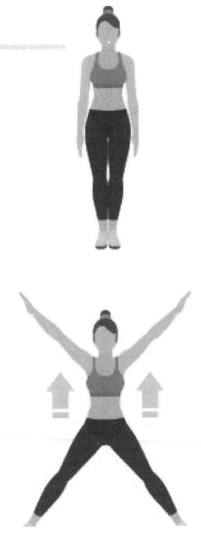

Press-Ups

Make sure your back is as straight as possible. And extend your arms as much as you can when you push your body up. Your overall posture will improve as a result of this exercise.

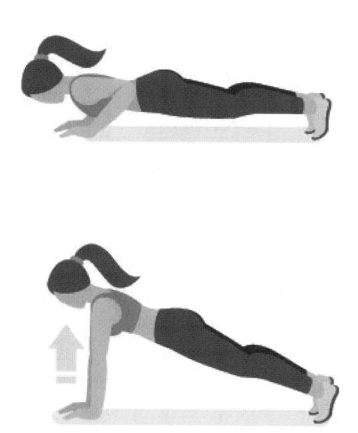

Alternate Leg Stretches

Stand up straight. Now bend both legs slightly and stretch your right leg out so that your left leg is half bent. Pull your left leg back and slowly stand up straight. Now switch legs and repeat the procedure until you've done 25 with each leg.

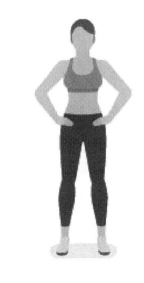

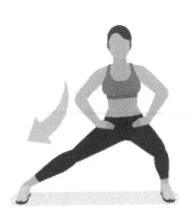

Stomach Crunches

Sit on your right side and rest on your right arm and elbow. Then put your fingers hand on the left side of your stomach. Cross your left leg over your right. Now lift your arm off the floor and slowly sit up, all the while concentrate on the stomach muscles. That is where you should feel the tension. Then return slowly to your original position.

Now repeat the exercise whilst sitting on your left side. Alternate until you've done 25 on each side.

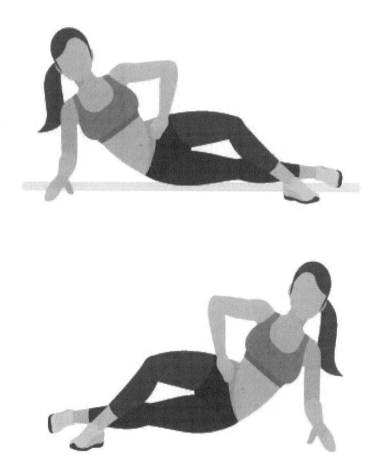

Alternate Leg Raises

Lie on your back. Lift your left leg so that your foot is about 18 inches off the floor. All the while keep your leg as relaxed as possible and concentrate on keeping the tension in your upper leg and backside.

This area should act as a pivot for your leg to move. Make your leg feel like a dead weight.

Now repeat the process with your right leg. Then left again until you've done 25 with each leg.

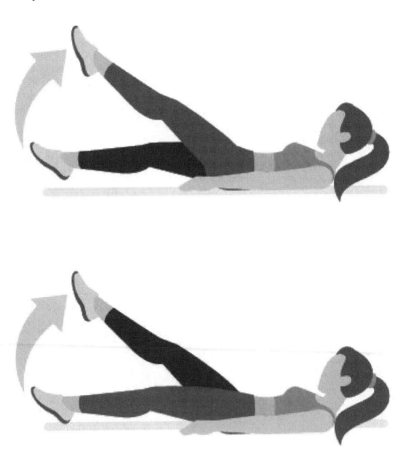

Cycling

Lie on your back and raise your legs. Then as if you were riding a bike, cycle with your legs in the air. Time yourself and do 25 seconds at a speed that is comfortable for you.

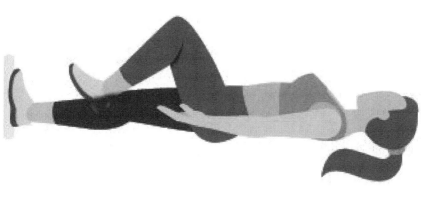

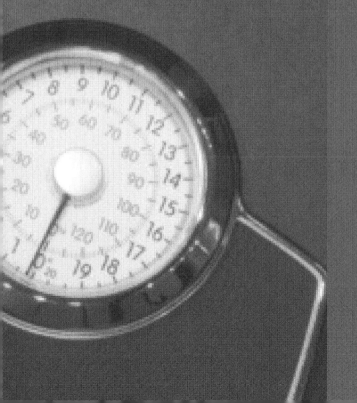

chapter **6**

Your Ideal Weight

n my experience most people choose a random
figure as their ideal weight. If you have a vague or
arbitrarily chosen goal in mind you've far less chance
of success.

Having a size of clothing that you want to fit into is better. But
let's be more specific.

First of all we need to determine how overweight you actually
are. Go to the online BMI weight calculator here:

http://www.nhs.uk/Tools/Pages/Healthyweightcalculator.aspx
Visit these links for US reader-friendly conversions:
http://www.metric-conversions.org/weight/stones-to-
pounds.htm
http://www.metric-conversions.org/length/feet-to-inches.htm

Let's use a fictional character as our example: meet Marie. She's
33, 5' 5" height and weighs 11 stone (182 lbs). Using the BMI
weight calculator, Marie is at least 3 lbs overweight.
Losing those 3 lbs would be sufficient to put Marie into the
Healthy Weight category. But chances are that Marie wants to
lose more weight than that. Marie decides to aim for a weight in
the middle of the Healthy Weight category: 9 stone 7 lbs (133
lbs).

It is up to you to decide on the weight you want to aim for. My
advice for a healthy man or woman is to set your target at a
number in the middle of the Healthy Weight category.

Do you have any doubts about your physical health? Do you believe that you have a body type that the BMI index does not take into account?

Then my advice is to consult your physician so that you can determine an optimum target for your weight loss goal.

Also note that there are variables in Asian people relating to ideal weights. For further reading on this see

https://en.wikipedia.org/wiki/Body_mass_index

After taking the above into account, make a decision on the exact weight you want to reduce to. Keep that goal in mind. Write it on a sticky note and put it on your computer so that you see it all the time. Put a note in your wallet or purse that you refer to every day.

Do what it takes.

Because once you know where you're going, The Wine Drinker's Diet is your roadmap to achieving your ideal weight — and staying there.

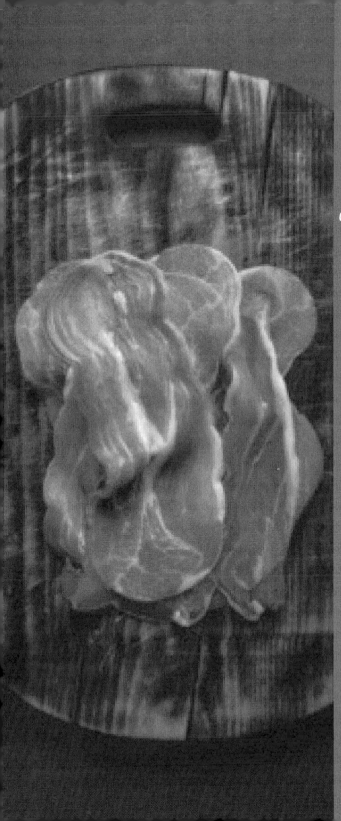

Level One: Fast Track To Rapid Weight Loss

In Chapter One I tell you how to prepare immediately before starting The Wine Drinker's Diet. But rather than go into Level One cold turkey, you should do some additional preparation beforehand too.

Cut down on caffeine as soon as you can

If you're used to a lot of caffeine you will inevitably feel tired when you cut it out of your diet.

It's not uncommon for us to go through most of our lives as caffeine addicts without being aware of it.

If you can reduce caffeine or get rid of it entirely before Level One, you'll be off to a head start.

Don't attack the food

Just because you're going on a diet, doesn't mean you have to go crazy before you start The Wine Drinker's Diet. Start to eat more healthily. Grill or steam your food. Don't fry it. Opt for white meat like chicken fillets or pork. Fish is an excellent source of lean protein too.

Clear the cupboards

Get rid of foods that you need to avoid. That means crackers, biscuits and sweets. Anything that needs no preparation will be easy temptation in the early stages of The Wine Drinker's Diet.

Most of the food you eat should need making before eating. That means less craving and more discipline. There's no getting away from it: you'll need some will power to make this diet work. But as you get used to it, The Wine Drinker's Diet will get a lot easier.

Stock up on low carb vegetables — carrots are great for snacks.

If you're taking your food to work, prepare it the night before.

Level One Menu
See the Food And Drink Table at the end of this book before preparing these dishes.

Day One

Breakfast
One boiled egg

Lunch
Three rashers of grilled bacon

Dinner
One skinless chicken fillet steamed or grilled with vegetables

Day Two

Breakfast
Porridge made with water or skimmed milk

Lunch
One skinless chicken fillet steamed or grilled and cut into strips

Dinner
Steamed or grilled vegetables and brown rice

Day Three

Breakfast

One scrambled egg with a teaspoon of olive oil or butter

Lunch

Steamed or grilled haddock

Dinner

Pork chop grilled with vegetables

Day Four

Breakfast

One boiled egg

Lunch

Three slices cold meat

Dinner

Two grilled sausages with vegetables

Day Five

Breakfast

Porridge made with skimmed milk or water

Lunch

One boiled egg

Dinner

Grilled steak with vegetables

Day Six

Breakfast
One egg omelette cooked with a teaspoon of olive oil or butter

Lunch
Smoked salmon

Dinner
Pork chop grilled with vegetables

Day Seven

Breakfast
Porridge made with water or skimmed milk

Lunch
Three x slices cold meat

Dinner
Two grilled sausages, three rashers bacon, one boiled egg

Drinks

Still or fizzy water
Fruit infusion teas
Decaffeinated tea and coffee

Snacks

Carrots
One egg extra per day

About The Level One Menu

See the Food And Drink Table which lists allowed food weight when necessary. This is particularly important for slow release carbs like brown rice and oats. If we're not accurate with measurements with carb-based food this can easily lead to plateaus or weight gain.

The weights apply to each individual serving, and are pre-cooked amounts — so weigh the food before it's cooked, not after.

You'll see that eggs crop up a lot in the Wine Drinker's Diet. The humble oeuf is your secret weapon! They're protein packed and very filling.

I've found that one egg is sufficient to keep me full till lunchtime on Level One. Another another egg around 1 pm and I'll be set till dinner.

And before I was on Level One of The Wine Drinker's Diet I routinely ate three rashers of bacon, two sausages and a slice of black pudding for breakfast. So if I can do it, so can you!

However, I realise that most people will want more variation in their diet than I had while I lost weight, so that's reflected in the Level One menu plan.

Always buy your bacon and sausages from a trusted local butcher. Strictly speaking we're avoiding processed foods. As bacon and sausages are processed, we want them to be the best possible quality. So avoid pre-packed supermarket bacon and sausages.

This doesn't apply to other meats, which will work out expensive if you always buy them from the butchers. Pre-packed supermarket meat is fine in most cases.

Always steam or grill food rather than frying it. Boiling it is fine too (though not as tasty!).

To steam cook salmon and vegetables for example, fill your steamer with about half an inch of water. Place the salmon and vegetables in the microwave. Then cook on full power until the salmon is cooked through. This is three - four minutes with most microwaves. Your food is now ready to eat. What could be simpler?

Garnish meat and fish with pepper and fresh herbs. If you need it lightly sprinkle on a small amount of salt too. Then finish off with a squeeze of lemon or lime juice.

Measurements aren't needed for most of the recipes. A handful of vegetables for example is sufficiently accurate. Serve meat in single portions; one chicken fillet, one pork chop and so on.

Throw away fat from meat before serving.

Try to stick to three meals a day.

If necessary, carrots and another egg make good snacks that should tide you over till lunch or dinner.

The meals on Level One are all basic and easy to prepare. That means you're getting used to good, simple, natural food. But I know basic food can get a bit boring after too long. Hang in there because we're going to switch it up a bit with more recipes and greater variation in Level Two.

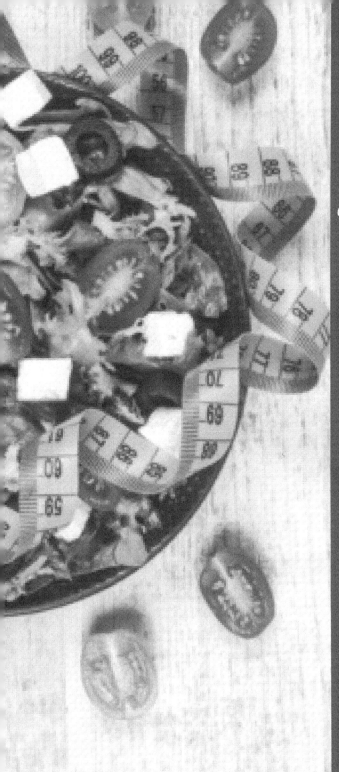

chapter **8**

Level Two: Maximise Your Dieting Success

Congratulations on making it this far! Now The Wine Drinker's Diet starts to get a little easier...

Level Two Menu

Day One

Breakfast

Bacon omelette
One egg, one rasher of bacon. Fry in bacon fat.

Lunch

Low fat or natural live yoghurt with carrot sticks
Five tablespoons of yogurt.

Dinner

Potato and cheese.
Microwaved or baked potato with melted mozzarella cheese

Day Two

Breakfast

Cheese Omelette
One egg, feta cheese. Fry in a teaspoon of olive oil or butter.

Lunch

Cold meat platter
Five slices of cold meats.

Dinner
Lamb chop and grilled vegetables

Day Three

Breakfast
Mixed fruit and yoghurt
Two slices each from three different fruits. Serve with two tablespoons of natural live or low fat yoghurt.

Lunch
Feta Cheese Salad
Use eight small cubes of Feta with vegetables.

Dinner
Grilled lamb chop with vegetables

Day Four

Breakfast
One boiled egg, one grilled sausage

Lunch
Greek salad
Eight small cubes of feta with olives and a green salad.

Dinner
Chicken and vegetables
Roast chicken leg or breast, oven cooked with vegetables.

Day Five

Breakfast

Two sausages

Lunch

Goat cheese and vegetables
Eight small cubes of goat cheese with the vegetables.

Dinner

Grilled steak and vegetables

Day Six

Breakfast

Bacon omelette
One egg, one rasher of bacon. Fry in bacon fat.

Lunch

Cold meat platter
Five slices of cold meats.

Dinner

Aubergine and cheese
Cook in the oven or microwave. Sprinkle one tablespoon fresh grated parmesan cheese onto the aubergine after cooking. Melt mozzarella onto the aubergine for a lower cost alternative.

Day Seven

Breakfast
Mixed fruit and yoghurt
Two slices each from three different fruits. Serve with two tablespoons of natural live or low fat yoghurt.

Lunch
Edam cheese salad

Dinner
Two sausages, two rashers of bacon

Snacks
Two tablespoons natural live or low fat yoghurt
One slice of cold meat

Level Two reintroduces low fat cheese. Only eat cheeses that are naturally low in fat, not cheeses with reduced fat. So Weight Watchers Reduced Fat Cheese is off the menu, mozzarella cheese is fine. For each meal use two thin slices of cheese.

Buy natural live yoghurt if you can. The lower end supermarkets do not normally stock natural live yoghurt. Buy low fat as a cheaper alternative, or when natural live yoghurt is unavailable. Thick Greek natural live yoghurt is one of the tastiest yoghurts available. Always buy plain yoghurt.

Sticking to the menu choices I've provided you with will result in weight loss. But you'll no doubt want to vary your choices too. Just consult the list of permitted food on the left hand side of your Level One Food guide when you need inspiration.

And if you particularly like one meal for breakfast, stick to it. Have it for lunch too if you like!

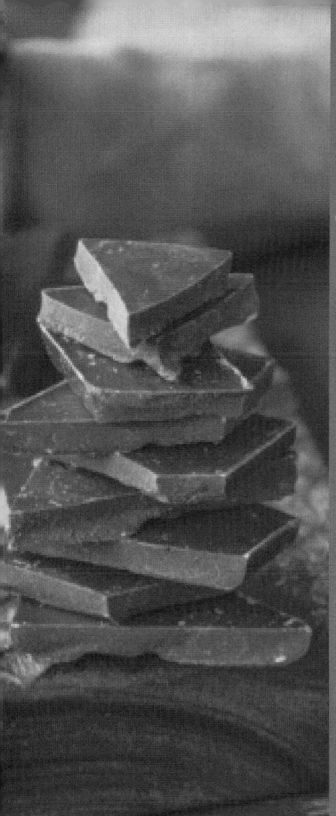

chapter **8**

Level Three: Keeping The Weight Off For Good

Level Three is for when you've reached your optimum weight. You can cheat a little, but not all the time. The closer you stay to real food the better.

You are basically continuing with Level Two but allowing yourself a little leeway. Watch your weight and your waistline and you'll be fine.

If you want a pack of potato crisps for example, choose the plain option. Stay away from flavoured additives. And have them for lunch. Don't have them instead of lunch.

Perhaps you'd like a bar of chocolate instead of your usual breakfast. If so choose plain high cocoa content chocolate. This is far less processed than most chocolate, so for a once in a while treat, these relatively unprocessed chocolates are the ones to go for.

I'd particularly advise caution with any food that includes sugar. If you had a sweet tooth before you began The Wine Drinker's Diet there's a chance that your sugar addiction could return. So make sure any sweet snacks are taken only on rare special occasions rather than frequently.

If you'd like some crackers to go with a couple of slices of cheese, choose crackers with just a few ingredients rather than a lot of E numbers. Cream crackers are a good choice, and are also low in carbohydrates. Again these must be a substitute for one of your meals, not an addition.

You can enjoy high carb content vegetables like potatoes and parnsips in moderation. Roasted, steamed, grilled or boiled are the best cooking methods for vegetables and meat alike.

And if you find that you've put on a few pounds then go right back to Level Two and stick to it until you're back to your ideal weight.

If you go completely overboard then start as soon as possible on Level One again. You've already reached your target weight once. With a bit of effort you'll easily do it again.

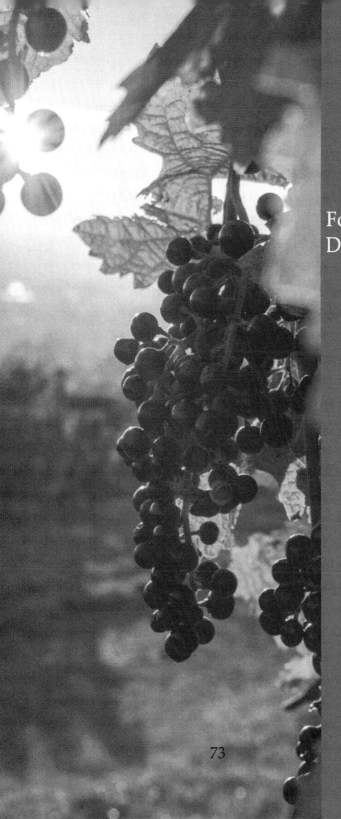

Food And
Drink Table

Level One:
Allowed

Alcohol

One of these choices per night with two dry nights. You can vary them through the week — so you might have wine one night and switch to spirits the next night for example.

Wine And Sparkling Wine:

One - three 6 oz. glasses during the evening, five times a week:

Red Wine

Rosé Wine

Dry White Wine

Champagne

Prosecco

Spirits

One - three 35 ml measures during the evening, five times a week. Mix with still or fizzy water.

Brandy

Irish whiskey

Gin

Rum

Scotch whisky

Tequila

Vodka

Light Beer

One - two bottles a night, with two dry nights a week.

I have listed light beers by brand and name because there are a few light beers that contain almost as many carbs and calories as a standard beer. Here are the ones I recommend:

Amstel Light
Budweister Select
Budweister Select 55
Busch Light
Coors Light
Corona Light
Labatt Aspens Edge
Michelob Ultra
Miller Light
Miller 64
Milwaukee's Best Light
Molson Ultra
Natural Light
Rolling Rock Green Light
Schmidt's Light

Meat

Remove fat and skin from meat before eating. Lean white meat is always the preferred option. However all other non pro-cessed meats are permitted too.
Sausages high quality, from your trusted local butcher only.
Bacon, as above.

Fish

Eggs

Herbs
A teaspoon sprinkled on food.

Vegetables
Asparagus
Bean sprouts
Broccoli
Cabbage
Carrots
Cauliflower
Celery
Cucumber
Leeks
Lettuce
Mushrooms
Onion
Spinach
Tomato
Turnips

Fruit
Lemon juice, 1/2 teaspoon only for seasoning
Lime juice, as above

Water
Still or fizzy

Seasoning

Vinegar, one teaspoon only
Olive Oil, one teaspoon only
Salt, A pinch only

Level One:
Not Allowed

Alcohol
Beer (non light)
Liquors
Flavoured drinks
Sweet cocktails

Bread And Grain Products

Cereal

Fruit
All other fruit except those that are listed in the Allowed category.

Juices

Processed Fish Products

Processed Meat
Except sausages and bacon from butchers.

Sauces

Smoothies

Sugar Based Products

Level One For A Week Plus

If you stay on Level One for more than a week, supplement any two of your meals per week with one of the following

Fruit
1/2 Grapefruit
One Mandarin Orange
One Satsuma

Level Two:
Allowed

These are in addition to the Allowed/Not Allowed food and drink on Level One.

Naturally Low Fat Cheese
Edam
Gouda
Cottage Cheese
Mozzarella
Feta

Yoghurt
Plain Low Fat
Plain Natural Live Yoghurt

Potatoes
Baked only. Add cottage cheese, yoghurt or melted low fat cheese.

Level Three... And A Final Word

Avoid food that you crave on Level Three. Aim to enjoy everything in moderation and stick to unprocessed fresh food.

Always read the ingredients list when you buy pre-packaged items. Look out for sugar and sugar under a different name (sucrose, fructose, dextrose are all sugars). Avoid also chemicals and E numbers.

Stay away from food that you've previously had a craving for. Monitor your weight carefully. If you start to put on weight, go back to Level One again.

No food is strictly forbidden when you reach Level Three, but you should proceed with care and monitor your weight so that you don't start to put on the pounds again.

In the introduction to this book I told you about my difficulties with dieting. After formulating and following The Wine Drinker's Diet those struggles are in the past for me.

Now I've reached my ideal weight. I stay there pretty much all of the time. And if I put on a couple of pounds over the holidays? A week on Level One puts me right again.

Changing my life for good with The Wine Drinker's Diet has been an amazing experience.

Just think: very soon you could be saying exactly the same thing.

Your Partner In Weight Loss Success

Pete.

Index

cheese, mozzarella 65, 67, 68, 81
cheese, reduced fat 68
cheese. parmesan 67
chemicals 82
chicken fillet 58, 58, 62, 57
chicken, breast 66
chicken, leg 66
chicken, skinless 37
chocolate 22, 71
chocolate, plain high cocoa 71
cocktails, sweet 79
coffee 38
coffee, decaffeinated 60
crackers 57, 71
crackers, cream 71
crisps 15
crisps 71
cucumber 77
cycling 43, 49
dairy 35
depression 30
detox 33
dextrose 82
diet, low carb 43
diet, low fat 37, 43
diet, pulse-based 36
diet, vegetarian 36
dinner 33, 58, 59, 60, 62, 65, 66, 67
doctor 23, 26
drinks, flavoured 79
e additives 71
e numbers 82
egg 16, 23, 24, 25, 36, 38, 58, 59, 60, 61, 62, 65, 66, 67, 77
exercise 23

Made in the USA
Lexington, KY
15 May 2019